SAS Survival Guide:

15 Prepper's Lessons You Should Know In Order To Survive In The Wilderness

Table of content

Introduction

There are many people around the world who love to pack a few essential items into a bag and head off into the wilderness. Some may simply be looking to travel the globe and experience new things; others may want to prove themselves and take on some of the harshest terrains known to man.

The truth is that the world is getting smaller, travel is actively encouraged and there are an abundance of opportunities to get out and see the world. Whilst this is an exciting opportunity and one which will create memories which will last a lifetime; it can result in you finding yourself in a survival situation.

Of course, people who go travelling, seeking adventure and who are prepared to travel to places that many others wouldn't dream of should be prepared. However, in reality many of these people will never have thought about the possibility of being stranded in the middle of nowhere. The experiences they have already had and their personalities may help them to make the most of the situation, and, with a little luck they will survive. In fact, it is better if they are prepared and have some basic equipment with them; it can make survival much easier.

It is important to realize that, even if you are not that adventurous a traveler, it is possible to become lost in the wilderness. Planes do crash and boats can sink; you can even just get lost in an incredibly heavy fog on moorlands. The wilderness may be different, but the result is the same; you are out of touch with civilization and need to survive on your own wits. You probably carry a cell phone but you may not be able to get a signal or it may be damaged, leaving you needing to survive and find your way home. Whilst these scenarios may seem farfetched for your everyday life; you never know what will happen each day, or on your next vacation. A little preparation will make all the difference if something ever did happen. Simply reading this book and carrying a few basic supplies can make a huge difference to your chances of survival.

If you should ever find yourself in this situation you must try to stay calm. The most important first step is to assess what items you have available. List every item mentally, or even on paper if you have some and a pen. Don't forget items such as shoelaces can be managed without and may be exceptionally useful for something else. If you know what you are carrying, then you will be aware of what may be adapted to each situation you come across. It is also important to consider what equipment anyone else has with you; or, if the worst has happened you will need to confirm what items are useful on anyone who has been killed by the incident. Equally, if you were in a vehicle or plane there may be useful equipment you can access; don't forget how important food and water are.

If you are fortunate enough to have a good collection of supplies, you will need a bag or some means of transporting it. A sheet can be dragged behind you, with the sides lifted up by making a hole in each corner and adding pieces of string, (or shoelaces, if you don't have any other string to hand.)

You must then assess the area you find yourself in. Depending upon how you have arrived in the wilderness may affect your next decision. If you are by a vehicle of plane and have some supplies, you may consider waiting with the transport. This may make it easier for rescuers to find you, but it may also make it easier for wild animals to find you. Taking a good look at the area you are in and the safety provided by you transport vehicle will help you decide where to stay; even if just for the first night.

This is the third important step; you must calculate the time and use this to help you make a decision. If you need to build a shelter and it is already starting to get dark, you may be better staying with the vehicle. If, however, you have all day it may be preferable to get away from the wreckage. Whichever option you decide upon you will then need to start thinking about how to survive; for as long as it will take for you to be either rescued or find your way back to civilization.

The tips in the next few chapters will help to make this possible.

Chapter 1 – 5 Tips to Ensure you Survive the Night

If it is already getting late in the day or you have no idea where you are and which direction to head in, then it is best to decide upon a suitable shelter and sort out your supplies; making sure you are ready to get up and get going the following day. A variety of modern pieces of equipment, such as a cell phone may not be able to put you in contact with your rescuers, but it can be put to other uses. Keeping your mind open will help you to survive; which is the one thing that really matters.

Shelter

To survive the night, you will need shelter from the elements. You may be able to locate a cave or rocky overhang which will protect you from any downpours. However, if you find a cave be careful it is not already being used by something else! If this is not an option, you should find a spot between two trees but where you are not likely to be hit by any falling object.

To create a basic shelter, you will need a log which is slightly longer than the distance between your two trees. Tie this log to the trees horizontally, you can use shoelaces, cord from a bracelet or even spare clothes to do this. Failing this you will need to find some vines or bendy sticks to secure it.

You will then need to put several more logs against the first one and a t a rough angle of forty five degrees to the ground. Then tie these logs on.

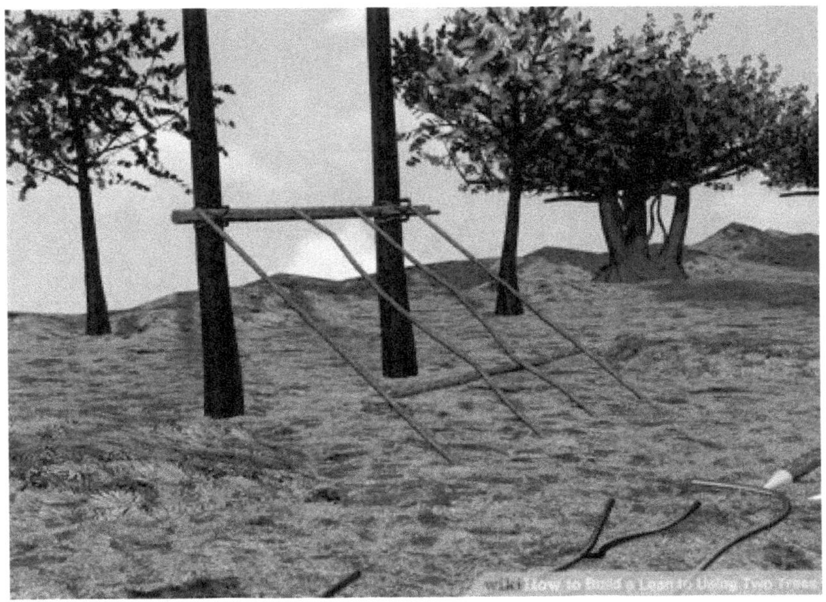

You should now add some branches going horizontal across the downward angle logs. Ideally these should be woven between the logs to help hold them in place.

Finally, you can cover the structure with leaves, pine branches with leaves on are excellent for this; they can also be used to create a soft flooring inside your lean to; helping you to be comfortable overnight. If you happen to have any tarpaulin you can just use this! Pine leaves or moss will help to insulate you from the ground; without them you will rapidly lose body heat.

If you have time you can continue the branches at each end of the shelter; leaving only the front edge open.

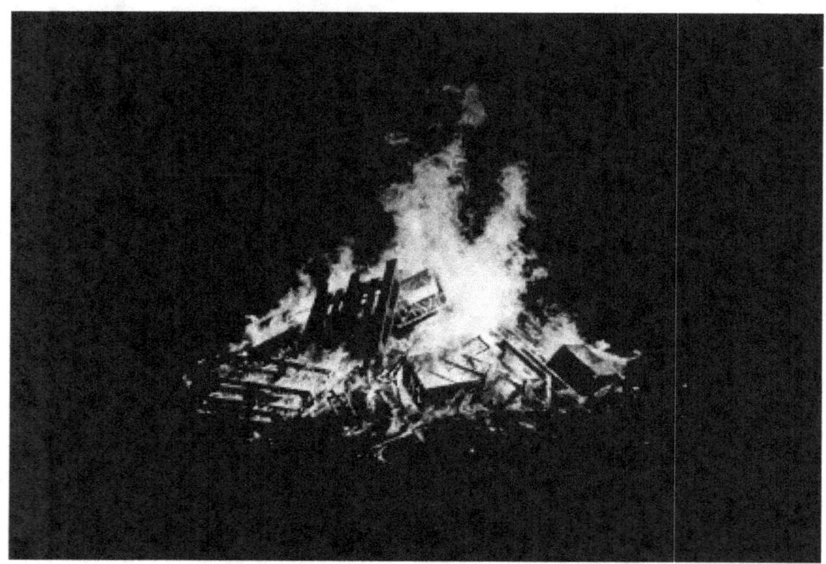

A shelter will keep you dry and help to keep you warm overnight. This is essential as you need to refresh yourself in order to remain focused.

However, you will also need a fire; this will help to keep you warm; especially if you have nothing to cover yourself with. It will also help to keep inquisitive animals at bay. To create a fire you will need some dry twigs, leaves and even dry moss if there is any to hand. A supply of dry branches will help to keep the fire burning throughout the night. You should be able to locate some wood in the wilderness, unless you are in the middle of the ice and snow.

To start your fire you must start by lighting the dry leaves, moss of small twigs. If you are not fortunate to have a lighter you can start the fire by using a pair of glasses to magnify the sun's energy. Alternatively, you can create a dip in a small piece of bark and find a piece of wood to use as a spindle. The idea is to spin this fast enough to cause friction against the bark and create a spark, lighting the moss or leaves. However, a spindle will quickly burn and blister your hands. Instead, create a make shift bow from a curved piece of wood and some string. You can then loop the string around the spindle and use a piece of wood to hold the spindle in place. This piece of wood should be in your left hand and the bow in your right, unless you are left handed. Moving the bow back and forth rapidly will quickly get your fire started.

Warmth

Having established your shelter and a fire you are well on your way to surviving the night. Although you may feel hungry and thirsty this is not something that you necessarily need to concern yourself with until the morning. Obviously if you have plenty of daylight left you can address this issue immediately using the tips in the next chapter.

It is also important to consider any injury you have. Stopping bleeding and wrapping any wound will help to prevent you from getting an infection.

Finally, depending upon the climate where you are stranded, you may wish to consider how cold it will get. An adequate supply of wood will keep your fire burning and a thick layer of moss will help prevent you from losing heat to the ground. If time permits you can locate additional moss or pine leaves to cover yourself with whilst you sleep. This will make you more camouflaged to wild animals and keep you warmer. This is important as your survival depends on getting adequate sleep; staying warm will help you to sleep.

Weapon

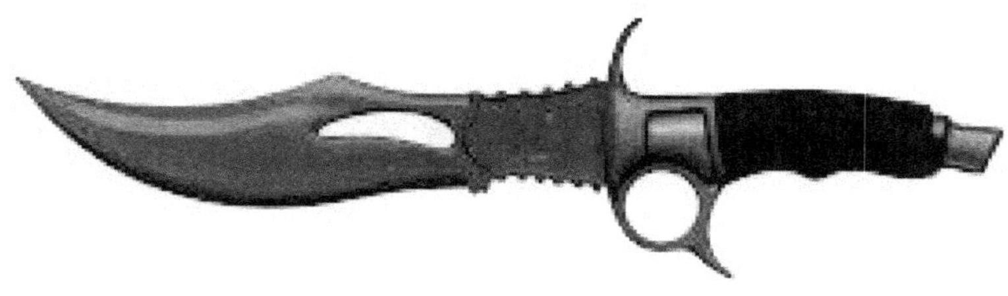

It is best to purchase a good pocket knife now and carry it with you at all times. In fact, being fully prepared should also include making a bracelet or key chain from paracord to give you a good length of strong string if you are ever stranded in the wilderness.

A knife, or alternative weapon, can help you stay alive if a curious animal strays to close or becomes a threat. If you do not have a knife the best alternative is to fashion a bow from a curved piece of wood and a piece of string. Arrows can be made from a sturdy twig and you will have something with you to help make a tip; such as a key or even a bank card.

Rescue Plan

Finally, as you settle for the night you must calm your mind. Focus on the images that make you feel comfortable and on what you will do when you get back to civilization. Once your mind is calm you will be able to consider the best route forward in the morning. The speed by which you are found will depend on how you have come to be stranded and who knows of your whereabouts. If it is likely that a rescue party will be dispatched quickly then your plan should revolve around how to attract their attention when you see a helicopter flying overhead. The fire will help; logs laid out as an SOS in a clearing are also likely to be seen. If rescue is likely to be within a few days then you are best advised to make yourself as comfortable as possible and stay put; surviving on food and water near your shelter.

However, if it is unlikely that a rescue party will be forthcoming you should use this period; when you are rational and clear thinking to decide on your best course of action. The direction you should head in will be defined by where you believe the closest civilization to be. Any plan should consider the distance you can travel, your current physical condition and the supplies you have. If you need to travel towards safety you may need to create shelter and a fire every night; this can be tiresome and limit the distance you can travel; you must consider this when devising your plan.

It may seem like a funny thing to be considering as you attempt to survive your first night, but, having a plan will give you focus and direction. This will help to prevent you from panicking and make the difference between surviving or not.

Chapter 2 – 5 Tips to Help you Find Food & Drink

Having created the right situation to survive the night, or even having survived it, you will now need to consider food and water. A human body can survive for weeks without food; however, you will struggle to survive more than a few days without water. Finding these and not being picky about what you eat, is essential to ensuring your keep your strength up and keep heading in the right direction.

Running Water

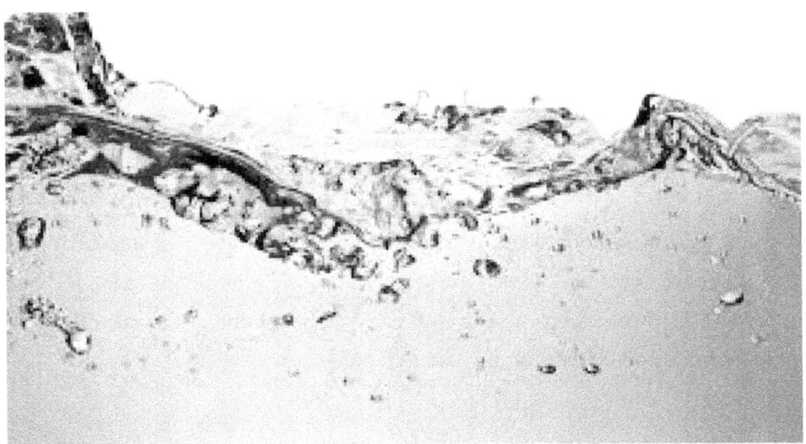

The best option for water is to find a stream or river. Not only is the water likely to be drinkable you may also be able to look at fishing in the water. Water tends to flow downwards; you will need to head downhill if you can and at the bottom of a valley there will often be water. A river can also be an excellent guide; following the direction of the flow will take you towards the sea and civilization. If you find a stream or river you should, ideally have something to collect the water in, putting your face to the water leaves you exposed to any wildlife in the area; be certain you are safe before you do this.

If possible, use a container of some description to carry water with you; either as you head for civilization or to keep at your base camp. You will not be able to confirm the cleanliness of the water but at this point anything is better than nothing!

If there is no stream then you may find a lake, a puddle, or even snow which can be melted. Alternatively, dig a hole in the ground and place a bowl in it, cover the hole with a piece of material and leave overnight. Condensation will collect in the cloth and drip into the bowl. You will also be able to wring the water out of the cloth.

There are several options when it comes to food and these will depend upon where you have become stranded and what is around you. At first glance you may see nothing which you can eat, but, as you become hungrier you will lower your expectations and settle for any sort of food!

Fishing

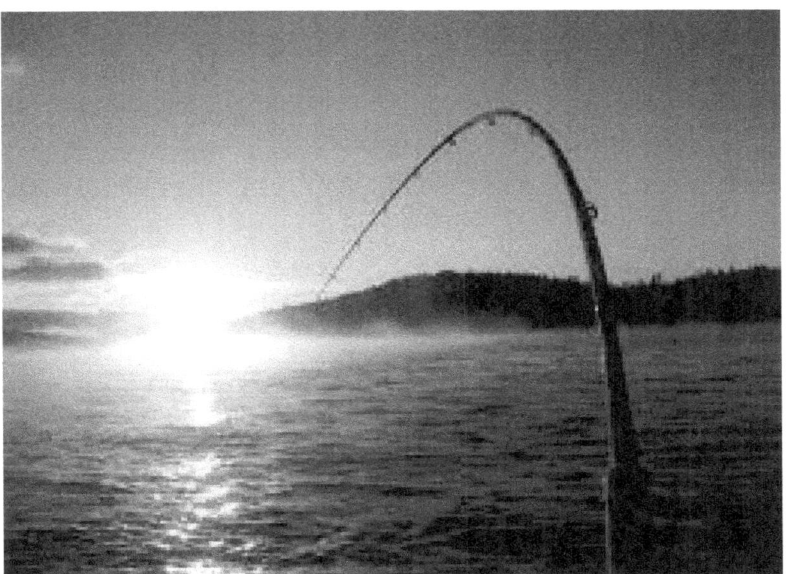

If you have found a stream or lake then there is a good chance that there will be some sort of fish in the water. The first step is to look in the water at the river bed, if possible, you may see crayfish or similar which you should be able to grab by their tail without any equipment. You can then cook these on your fire.

If you need to make a rod then any decent sized stick will do. Simply attach a piece of string on to the stick as a line and look for some grubs or worms near the water's edge.   You will need to tie these to your line and react quickly if something takes your bait; unless you happen to have a fish hook with you.

Alternatively you can use, if you have some, a fine piece of material as a net. Either hold this in the water or attach it to a stick in an attempt to catch a fish.

Finally, if you are planning on staying in one spot and waiting for rescue you may like to dig a small siding from the main stream.   Dig a pool and allow the water from the river to flow in.   Any fish which gets into the pool will be unable to jump back into the main river.

Grubs

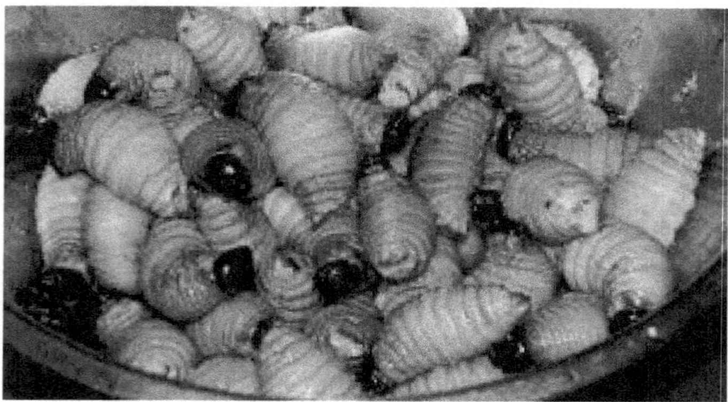

Once your hunger starts to take hold you will be able to contemplate eating grubs. They can be easily found by turning over rocks, especially in damp places.   These bugs may not be very large or appealing but they will be high in protein and fat;

which is essential to keep you moving. Grubs are generally easy to find and are abundant enough to provide a steady flow of food. They will taste better if you cook them, but if this is not an option then you will gain more nutrient value by eating them raw. Some of the best places to look for grubs are in decaying tree remains, inside a closed flower or even amongst the loose bark.

One huge advantage of eating grubs and insects is that it will not require a large amount of energy expenditure to locate them. This is an important consideration as you do not want to expend one thousand calories obtaining a five hundred calorie meal. When you cook your grubs it is best to wrap them in leaves, this will help to destroy any bacteria and make it easier for your body to digest the proteins.

Most bugs can be eaten, those which should be left alone are generally any which are covered in fur or have bright colored outer shells. These are defensive mechanisms and indicate poisonous bugs; equally, any bug which is happy to crawl in the open is likely to be poisonous.

Fruits & Berries

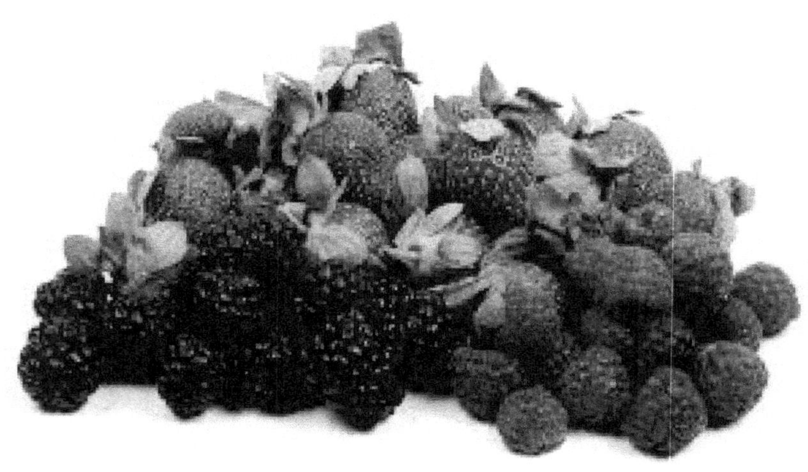

Ding upon where you have become stranded, you may find an abundance of fruits and berries on the trees and bushes around you. These will be easy to pick, nutritious and add some valuable liquid to your diet.

However, how do you know if a fruit or berry is safe to eat? The best course of action is to start studying fruits and berries now; you will then be sure of what is edible and what is not! Unfortunately, you may be stranded before you have time to complete your research. In this instance it is best to base your decision on whether to eat or not on the plant. Anything which looks prickly or dangerous should be avoided; as should anything with a milky sap. A plant whose leaves form in clusters of three should always be avoided and anything which looks similar to a fruit you know, but is not that fruit; should definitely be avoided.

If you are in doubt and can find no other food then it is best to taste a very small piece of the plant or fruit. If it has a soapy taste, or even seems bitter it is likely to be bad for you. If not, then, providing you have no ill effects within a few hours you should be able to eat more of them.

Birds Eggs

In general, it is safe to eat any bird egg, in fact, they can be quite tasty boiled in water and added to some gunk from the inside of a cactus. Cacti are one of the exclusions to the thorny outer but edible inner. The gooey mixture inside a cactus is very good for you and tastes fairly decent when boiled. Mix this with your egg and you will have a balanced meal!

If there are trees around you then the nests will generally be high up, this does not mean they are inaccessible! However, you will also find that there are plenty of birds which either lay their eggs on the floor or make a small hole to put them in. If you scout the floor while you walk you may see some.

Chapter 3 – 5 Tips to Help you Survive

Being stranded in the wilderness is frightening, the prospect of walking for days without knowing where you are going is scary; but the thought of going around in circles and never being found is terrifying! Even the most organized person in the world is highly unlikely to have a map and a compass on them when they become stranded. This means that you must look at other ways of ensuring you know which direction you are facing and which way you want to go. Thankfully there are a number of ways of making sure you are moving forward and heading the right way:

North

There are two ways of finding north. The first is at night time. If you look at the night sky you will see the big dipper; if you are unfamiliar with this star, then now is the time to teach yourself to recognize it. The two stars at the edge of the big dipper will lead you directly to the North Star; it will be above them and in a straight line with them.

If you need to find north in the daytime then it is best to locate a straight stick and sink it into the ground. Assuming the sun is out, you will instantly see a shadow, this points north.

Once you have located north you will be able to work out south, east and west. All you need to do then is decide which direction you wish to head in and stay heading that way; at least you will know you are making progress; not walking in circles. It is also worth remembering that the sun rises in the east; this will help to confirm your direction of travel.

Of course, knowing north is not only helpful if you wish to know which direction to travel in; it can also help you to calculate the time of day. This is important if you know it gets dark at six, you may wish to stop walking at three to create your camp for the night; it is important to never leave it too late to set up your camp.

Running Water

As already mentioned running water will take you in the general direction of the sea and civilization. Historically towns and villages were built on or near a water supply; this made one element of living easier!

Following a river is one way of almost guaranteeing you will find some form of civilization. However, you may find it difficult to stay near a river bank due to natural vegetation. This can make it exhausting making progress and increase the likelihood of injury.

Instead, you may decide this is a good opportunity to make yourself a raft and go with the river. Although this may take a little organizing, it will help you to make faster progress once you get going. A raft can be made by simply stacking several pieces of wood together and tying them to each other. You should also make sure you have a good long stick or two to help you steer while moving down stream.

You will not know what obstacles are ahead on the river so must take a cautious approach as much as possible. A lashed together in this fashion is not likely to last long in any rapids!

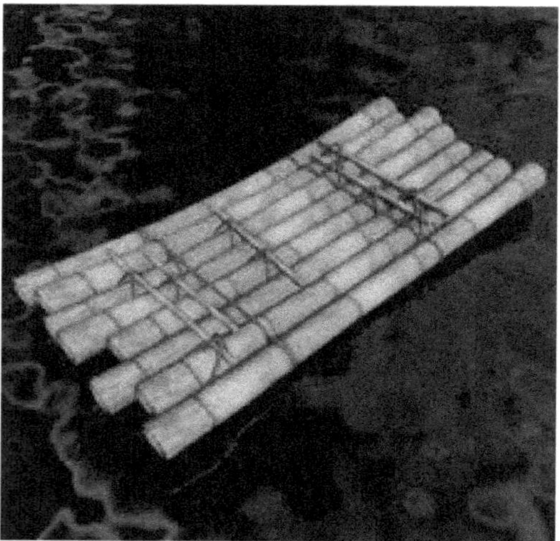

Essential equipment, such as your survival kit, a fishing rod and a few water containers can make your journey easier. These items should be tied to the raft to ensure they stay with you, even if the water gets choppy.

Water Filtering

The importance of water has already been stressed; without it you simply cannot survive. It is best to locate running water as this will be the least likely source of bacteria. Clear water should generally be okay whilst colored water or water with algae on should be avoided.

To prevent yourself from falling ill you need to ensure the water is clean; there are two ways of doing this. The first method is to boil the water; this will kill any bacteria in the water. You will obviously need to create your fire and have a suitable container for your water; it will need to be boiled for at least five minutes.

Alternatively you can filter the water. If you are in an area where there are birch trees you will be able to make a cone from the bark; this involves cutting piece of bark and shaping them into a cone shape; you will need to lash the bark together. You will also need to make sure there is a small hole at the bottom of the cone. You can then fill this cone with grass, followed by sand, then charcoal; repeat the filling process until the cone is filled to the top. You can then pour your water through this temporary filter and drink it!

You should be able to find charcoal from you first fire, or you may even be able to locate it as you explore the area around you. The sand, grass and charcoal will trap and kill any bacteria leaving you water which is as pure as possible in your situation.

Defenses

One of the things that many people forget in the wilderness is building perimeter defenses. Your shelter and a fire will help to keep animals at bay. However, it is better to have a warning that something is approaching rather than wake up face to face with an animal; no matter how big or small.

Perimeter defenses will also give you peace of mind. If you know that you need to listen for a specific sound then you can ignore the host of other sounds which you will hear in the wild. This will help you to sleep better.

In the wild, especially if you are travelling, you will not want to expend too much energy on a makeshift perimeter defense every night. The simplest way of doing this is to make a circle of brush small pieces of wood. This will make it difficult for any animal to cross and will give you warning as they'll be unable to get through without making a noise.

The longer you stay in one spot the stronger you will be able to make these defenses; fallen trees and large logs can be added to make a fence style perimeter. You perimeter should be just a few meters away from your shelter; providing enough room to warn you without trying to create too big an area and attracting more animals.

Signal

Finally, one of the most important aspects of being lost in the wilderness is being able to signal for help. Provided someone knows where you were going or what has happened, there will be search parties out looking for you. They may be able to follow a trial to find you, however, it is better to be able to signal them if you know they are there.

Fire is an excellent way of signaling rescue; people will see the smoke and, from above, the glint of the fire; helping them to locate you. Fires can even be used in the daytime; simply get a good fire going and create a frame around it. This will allow you to place foliage onto the fire without smothering it. By piling plenty of leaves and branches on you will almost smother the fire and create plenty of smoke.

Providing the sun is out you can use a mirror to reflect the sun into the air. This is a particularly effective way of getting a plane or helicopter to see you. The glinting mirror will catch their attention. A mirror can be made from anything you have which reflects the suns light; a belt buckle is an excellent example. This signal can be seen from a great distance by anyone flying and is extremely effective as well as easy to carry with you.

Conclusion

It is possible to survive in the wild with a small amount of planning and the ability to keep a clear and calm mind. One of the most important things which you need to be aware of is the importance of having a knife with you. This will make your survival attempt much easier as your knife can be used for a variety of different tasks. Whichever knife you choose must be comfortable to hold and one that you can easily carry around with you. Ideally you should carry your knife at all times but this may be easier said than done if you work somewhere which has security; they may not be comfortable with you having a knife and insist on keeping it at the reception during the day.

In fact; although the better prepared you are the easier you will find it to survive, the real solution to surviving in the wild comes from remaining calm. Every decision you make has the potential to put your life in danger. It is important to assess each situation calmly; if at all possible avoid making a rash decision and think through all the options. This will ensure you continue to head in the right direction and reduce any risk of a bad decision putting you in harm's way. When you are trying to survive in the wilderness you must consider every event that happens and make a decision based on what is most likely to help you survive.

There are several things you can do now to help assist you in this type of situation; should it ever happen;

- Buy yourself a good pocket knife; keep sharp and with you.

- Consider making yourself a survival bracelet or purchasing one which is ready made. These bracelets look stylish and are made of paracord; which is exceptionally strong and can be unraveled to provide you with plenty of rope in an emergency situation. You can even get bracelets which have flint in to help you start a fire in the wild.

- Practice; if you have a big enough garden to build a shelter or make your own fire then you should do so at home. If not, then you may wish to locate some woods nearby and practice making a shelter. It is worth checking before you try starting a fire in the woods; you do not want to burn the whole forest down!

Being lost in the wilderness is something that most people think will never happen to them. However, it can and does happen to anyone. Preparing yourself by reading this book, learning and understanding the tips and staying calm will help you to survive in any situation. No matter how difficult it may seem at first, there is always a way to survive; even if it means climbing inside a dead animal carcass to keep warm! It is essential to remember that everything you have with you could be useful in helping you survive.

FREE Bonus Reminder

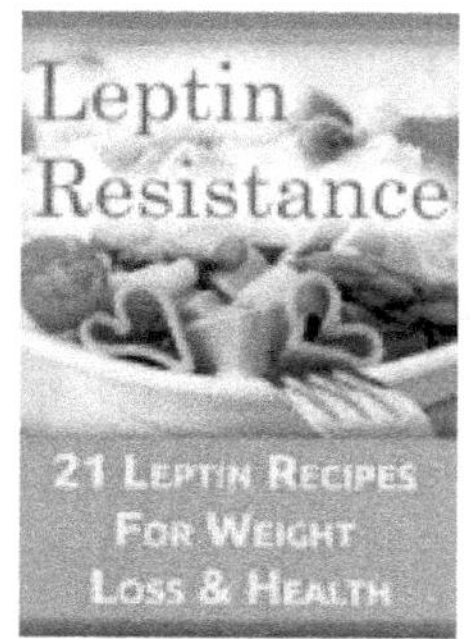

If you have not grabbed it yet, please go ahead and download your special bonus report *"Leptin Resistance. 21 Leptin Recipes For Weight Loss & Healthy Living"*.

Simply Click the Button Below

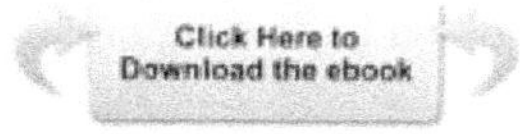

OR **Go to This Page**

http://easyweightlossway.com/free/

BONUS #2: More Free & Discounted Books

Do you want to receive more Free & Discounted Books?

We have a mailing list where we send out our new Books when they go free or with a discount on Kindle. Click on the link below to sign up for Free & Discount Book Promotions.

=> Sign Up for Free & Discount Book Promotions <=

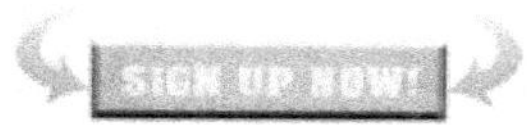

OR Go to this URL

http://zbit.ly/1WBb1Ek